Bald Bird

Kaye Howarth

Bald Bird

Contents

Bald Bird

Bald Bird

Bald Bird

Foreword

Hi, let me introduce myself, my name is Kaye.

It took me ten years to get round to actually face being able to put this book together, having remained roughly typed out, gathering dust under my telly in a black file.

It has taken another ten for me to get round to sharing it.

This book initially started off as a diary. For me to log small progress, or not, trials and tribulations that this diagnosis brings not only me but my family who also faced this with me. I apologise up front for writing as it comes out. I did consider changing and tightening things up, but I did write this twenty years ago and we change a lot in twenty years, given the chance.

Why now do I decide to pull this out and type up now?

Well I feel it might be useful for someone who may be just beginning this journey, someone who may be younger and with a family, who may perhaps find some comfort , know that I'm with them through their journey. Each journey is an individual one, but to know someone else has may have felt nearly every emotion you feel may help a little.

Bald Bird

Introduction

At the time of writing this I am thirty-three years young. Height 5.5ft, slimmish...was a Strawberry Blonde, do still have hazel eyes. Divorced for eleven years, and a single mum to my two gorgeous children Emily and George, both of whom are red heads! to my first husband.

I have recently remarried to Mick, a Prison Officer at HMS The Weare (A prison ship) who has two young daughters who stay with us every other weekend. Our family also includes a toothless Tortoiseshell cat called Pickles, who dribbles incessantly (she's 14 now) two rabbits, and two guinea pigs.

I work part time as a "Speech and Language Therapy Assistant", at Dorchester County Hospital, on the Adult Stroke unit, Hardy Ward. I love my job. Its only 15 hours a week; spread over three days, my old reliable car bravely takes me from Portland to Dorchester, and back again occasionally breaking down on Ridgeway Hill, which isn't fun. However... that's the least of my worries.

I am at the moment on sick leave. At present a "Bald bird", no hair. Just a rather good NHS wig style called Linda. I don't wear this locally, just a woolly hat, on brave days I don't bother to wear anything- my neighbours hail me in the street as "Sinead" that is as in O'Conner, the singer... I don't mind.... I'm bald. Last year I found a Breast Lump, I have Cancer. I'm scared.

Cancer changed my life, actually for the better, never before have I appreciated so much, the sweet (sometimes not so sweet) smell of my children's skin.

Bald Bird

Relished and resented the kindness of my fellow human beings at the time of my incapacity. I have been given a lesson to appreciate the day I'm in; something I never really did before, usually planning years ahead.

Bald Bird

A letter for Bert

I find I am beginning to have a relationship with my new lump. My fingers have taken on an obsession.

Just like a jealous partner, they keep checking that you're there. Of course, you're still there aren't you Bert?! One hopes that as with an old boyfriend who's bugged the crap out of you, has hopefully picked up the vibes that he's not wanted anymore. Has used incentive...and left, gone disappeared, just before the nasty, messy, screaming stage.

But you're still here. I shall call you "Breast Lump" Bert, seeing we are now- so to speak attached through my left breast. Just you know this though Bert, I hate you, and I hate all you've put me through. In a weird way though Bert, you have made me pull my life together, I appreciate the new insight you have gained me into how precious my life is.

Never again will I take for granted the sweet smell of my children's skin. The warmth of a hug with my husband, laughing with my mother on the phone, chuckling at naughty jokes emails sent by my best friend Annie, or the human kindness of the people who surround me.

So, Bert, it's just you and me, let the battle begin....

Bald Bird

A Definite Lump

My heart begins to pump so fast; I think it will explode through my ribs. Whistling sounds ring in my ears, the bath I sit in has no warming me, the bathroom walls zoom in.

"No God Please...not me!"

My hand moves around my left breast, I'm physically shaking, breath leaves my body in rapid bursts, any second I feel I will pass out. Stomach constricting, I mentally order myself to explore the outer perimeter of my left breast, once more.

There is definitely a pea size lump.

"You bastard, you bloody shitty bastard!" Life I meant. I had only just got mine, at the age of 32, in order, and then bugger me if it doesn't turn round and kick you in the teeth, just as you start to relax.

It's funny, but at that moment my life flashes before my eyes, photographic form

Snap! Me as a baby, lying in a huge pram, merrily sucking on my toes (no chance of that nowadays) oblivious to the surrounding wood pigeons cooing, and the glorious sunshine in the cloudless blue sky.

Snap! Mum and I, me as a gawky, skinny teenager, with stupid bunches sticking out of strawberry blonde hair, standing on top of some hill in Torquay, with a parrot (the photographers) glaring menacingly into my trusting eyes.

Snap! Karyn my best friend and I, both hormonally charged sixteen-year-olds, at a local photo booth, pulling faces, rushing out after being blinded by the flash of bulb. Unendurable three-minute wait for the four pictures to slide down the slot, self-conscious now, of the people guaranteed to turn up right behind you, as the photos slide down....

Snap! First love Barry, motorcyclist, had a Moto Guzzi 50cc, later had a sporty three-wheeler car, orange and black, had to push start it one day...

Snap! First husband, Weymouth Registry Office, children later, Emily first, then George both inheriting my red hair. Photos post-divorce.

Me and the kids in our new house, new friends, the children's, and mine. Parties, first days at school, crisp new uniforms...Christmases, learning the skills of balance on first bikes.

Snap! Present. Mick and I getting married at Thorn bury Castle 21.08.99 Bristol. George my son Best man, in top hat and tails. Emily my daughter, Chief Bridesmaid. in a golden off the shoulder gown. Our Stepdaughters their two little cousins and my niece blew across the resplendent lawns in white dresses, reminding me of Dandelions being blown gently in the warm summer breeze.

Lastly but no means least our young Pageboy, who gave me my lucky horseshoe. My wonderful grandparents Betty and Lesley, celebrating also on that day their 45th Wedding Anniversary. Photo with my Bouquet! Sob!

I HOPE AND PREY THAT I WILL MAKE OUR FIRST! AM I GOING TO DIE?

Bald Bird

Mum

It's at times like these that I thank god I have a fantastic relationship with my mum. Once the children were in bed, bribed with various goodies to help them on their way (as all good mothers know what to provide for a child free zone) I dial my mother's phone number.

Now my mum is a real character, she is classy, funny and has an inner strength that I have never met before, or am likely to meet again, she raised me alone from a young and tender age, and it was a struggle for her, but she did it!

"Hello!" sang a happy female voice. "Hi mum..." sniff...sob

"Okay hun...wots up then...?" her voice soft.

Sob. Sniff... "hi Mum, I've got another lump...!" (I had had a previous lump, which turned out to be a cyst, aspirated 12 months ago) Sniff...sob.

I then spent the next hour on the phone, with her telling me to make the Doctor's appointment the following morning. I said I would, she said she would pay for me to go private if necessary.

We end the conversation with her making me laugh, can't remember what she said, but it did the trick for the moment.

Mum says all will be ok, like a good girl I believe her, mums don't lie about such things, she says we had covered this ground before with the Cyst, and that was all ok. We say goodnight and after promising to phone her tomorrow evening. Having made the GP appointment, would see what the next steps would be.

I replace the receiver slowly, look around to Mick who stands behind me, and shrug.

Bald Bird

The following morning, I give breakfast to bleary eyed children. Pack lunch boxes and fill juice bottles to the brim. Gym Kit retrieved from airing cupboard for George.

The children feed rabbits, guinea pigs, and toothless cat Pickles.

I wave goodbye to their burdened backpacks as they disappear slowly up the hill merging with other backpacks of various sizes and colours. It is 8.45am, I make coffee, and get pen and paper. Watch the News for ten minutes, then pick up the phone and call Doctors.

The Receptionist listens to me, and my symptoms. Seeing it is a Monday, and you normally have to wait for an appointment, unless your head is hanging of your shoulders, I am warmly surprised by the efficiency of the young Receptionist who tells me to come in today at the end of Surgery."" Due to the circumstances Kaye, we would like to see you as soon as possible, so see you this evening." This is a command I agree with.

Bald Bird

The Appointment

"Kaye", the Nurse Practitioner calls me to her surgery. I sit down; give previous medical history, including the Aspiration of the Cyst in the same breast, this time last year.

She smiles encouragingly, in doing so I relax…a bit. As requested, I now lie down on the examination couch, disrobed to my waist. (Once you have given birth this is a ride in the park.)

The doctor gently examines both my breasts and confirms there is indeed a lump apparent in my left breast. Referral is then made for the Breast Clinic, which is held at Dorchester Hospital, Tuesdays, and Thursdays. Fourteen days wait at the most for my appointment. God bless the NHS. She lets me get dressed in privacy, and when leaves wish me gently "Good luck!"

At home Mick is waiting for me; I tell him all that was said.

"The return of the Cyst!" Mick smiles cynically" Sounds like the title of a horror film," We cuddle and laugh, sort of……

Okay', I'll level with you inside my head at that moment I'm thinking, will I live to see my children grown? Have I got Cancer? Is it in my hips? Bones? Liver? Kidneys, how much of my organs can they remove before the consultant says," That's all we can do for you?"

How the hell do I keep myself and my family going until I receive my appointment? Patience just isn't my strong point, nor is relying on others for information, which now I have to do, and wait for.

Everyone sees me carrying on, whilst I write Christmas Cards, (Christmas 1999) send my children on various postage missions, and drink Whisky (in moderation) with my husband in the evenings when the babes are safe asleep. We play Chess to stop me thinking about "It", we wrap Christmas pressies.

It's funny, but as word spread around my street of my predicament(although I hasten to add, I do not even feel ill, just run down) a support network begins to grow around me, friends I had lost contact with get back in touch, telling me of various members who had pulled through...I drink in positivity. Neighbours who are nodding acquaintances (due to busy work schedules etc) pop in with flowers, homemade biscuits for the kids, which are eaten rather quickly!" Homemade cakes, and Carol pops in from across the road for a coffee now and again. Offers of babysitting flood in, for as and when needed.

Bald Bird

What do I tell the kids?

Throughout this emotional turbulent time, Ems and George are aware of my health; they are given minimal but honest bit of information, saying basically I had a lump in boob that needed checking out. Although at this point other family members stepped in giving them support.

Emily carries on being a teenager, acting hormonally; she hasn't quiet reached that point woman hood yet, but likes to keep up appearances. George continues with his Play station Games, climbing and moving up Levels with his lifelong friend Sean, occasionally they can be seen on frequent fridge raids/ raiding the kitchen for sustenance.

I spend the majority of the weekend with mum, who truly brilliant, she's so scatty and makes me and the children laugh, we eat loads, lay by her fire, kids bicker and argue...normality, I had almost forget. Mum has offered the children to spend the night with her. A wonderful treat that usually happens every other weekend. As I can only sleep properly in my own bed I go home. Knackered and home. The phone rings, it's my Uncle Danny, quells my ensuing fears of up and coming appointment, we say goodbye. Mick phones that evening; he is having his children at his mums in Evesham. We play on the phone, arguing about who loves who the most, I let him win, cos he's better at arguing than me, the conversation ends. I place down the receiver.

The house at this moment feels very, very empty.

Bald Bird

Working week and Supportive work colleagues

It is Monday, I go to work at Dorchester Hospital, and I have spoken with my boss (and friend) Natalie, the Speech Therapy Team Leader. (I'm lucky in working in the caring profession,).

She makes me a coffee; I gather my thoughts.

We sit down for a coffee with Claire, another Speech therapist in the office.

I tell them all that has happened. They are supportive, Natalie suggests perhaps it would be an idea for Claire to accompany me to appointment; I am relieved, truthfully...because...

1. Mick travels to Bristol every other weekend to maintain contact with his girls.

2. It would take the pressure off him.

3. Claire has breasts

4. I can talk openly without fear of frightening her, and others at work.

5. I can tell them how shit-scared I am really.

Yes please I say, they give me a hug.

Claire and I then go to the Adult Stroke Unit to begin our day's work, as a word of advice to anyone who can manage this, work is a great distraction and anchorage, intermittently thoughts muscled their way my head, but I concentrated hard on my patients. I wondered what they would think if they knew what was going on in my life. Looking at the other staff, questioning myself, as to who else could possibly be going through an illness I didn't know about?

Bald Bird

Natalie keeps in close contact with me, telling me she had informed the Head of the Department of my condition. Thanks Nat you're a star, because sometimes just having to tell one more person can really do you in, especially at work.

Days tick away, work, children, washing, cooking.

I find through the ensuing days that I am beginning to have a relationship with my new lump, my fingers begin to take on an obsession, just like a jealous partner, I keep checking that you're there...of course you're still there aren't you Bert!.

Bald Bird

Seems like a lifetime

Two weeks isn't really a long time, but it's like anything. Waiting for exam results, waiting for a reunion, it seems a lifetime. Mick does his best in being positive; he spoils me and tries to take my mind of things.

Emily and George continue in their childhood.

People carry on with their everyday life, normality.

I'm jealous of their uncomplicated lives, don't they know I could be dying? Don't they know my children could be left without a mother???

I'm so angry at this blow life has given me.

I hate this life. I hate this bloody Cancer. I love life and want to live forever. I want to see my children grow into adulthood. I want to see Emily and George graduate, go to the Prom, college, get married. I want to have Grandchildren sit on my knee. I bargain with God, "Please God just give me ten years to see my children safely grown".

I look down at the kitchen floor; Pickles our cat is meowing pitifully at my feet, looking up at me lovingly I feel she is picking up on my emotional state, I then notice the cat flap has been shut.

I want the cat not to have peed on the kitchen floor.

Bald Bird

Watching the letter box

I find I am not sleeping at all, I'm getting grumpy with the children, and the entire universe. Busying myself over the next few days with all the household jobs. Trying hard to remain normal.

I go out and clean the rabbits in the howling, windy rain, and look up at the sky and shout... "Why me. What the hell have I done!" my words are dragged out of my mouth and thrown away to the grey skies.

Two sets of eyes look at me, with soft twitching noses.

Molly a grey long haired bunny turns to Toby, a pure white (I rescued him from the local pet shop as no one wanted him, he sways like a head banger, (some neurological problem) with pink eyes, and ignore me. The Guinea pigs squeak, and huddle in their straw refusing to even acknowledge the strange noisy human (would of course be different if a carrot was involved,) outside their warm domestic hutch.

I slop about with clean straw and hay, making them comfortable they do not feel like coming out today, although they have total freedom to run in the garden.

My hands are numb as I change the water feeders. So is my brain from thinking about it. "Cancer, the IT in my TIT", I think this and laugh to myself.

Kath my elderly next-door neighbour is emptying her bins, shakes her head sadly. Kath must think I've finally lost it, I say this to Pickles our toothless tortoise shell cat who has jumped into the rabbit hutch with Molly and Toby, who grumble, hiss and cuddled up anyway.

Bald Bird

I go inside, to the kitchen. I need hot coffee to warm my frozen hands.

Turning after flicking the kettle on, a large white letter drops through our letter box, silently landing on our" WELCOME" doormat.

This is the referral, I know it...It is, I'm right. Opening the letter with shaky hands read I have an appointment in two weeks' time...and My Consultant will be the same one who aspirated my Cyst last year. I am lucky, he is brill.

I stand motionless letter in hands, in my green wellies, straw in hair, and cry.

Bald Bird

The Referral

Having finished my work shift, I clamber down the hospital stairs, my energy level right now feels strangely low, and I feel totally drained. To keep my energy level up I find I have to eat every two hours, eating makes my jaw ache, and I seem to be finishing my meals long after everyone else.

I meet with Claire in our office; we discuss patient notes, and ideas in helping patients, relevant information. Then we discuss what we did at the weekend, and various middle of the range chit chat.

The time has arrived for my appointment at the Breast Clinic. Claire and I gather ourselves, my heart begins to speed up.

"Are you sure you don't mind coming?" I'm now feeling rather apprehensive to say the least; I know Claire won't let me down though I ask any way.

"Come on sweetie," Claire takes charge, and leads me to the door, downstairs across the passage, through another door. We have arrived; we turn right into the Breast Clinic.

The receptionist smiles warmly acknowledges my name firstly verbally, then checks out my NHS id badge, which after sitting down I remove swiftly and put in bag.

The Breast Clinic is fairly quiet, then it is early-1.45pm .Come 2.00pm the clinic   swells with woman of all age's partners, and children, and a few men patients, this is not just a female disease I remind myself. Claire squeezes my hand reassuringly. I'm embarrassed .as my palms are now damp and clammy; Claire doesn't seem to have noticed.

Bald Bird

My name is called by a cuddly Blonde Nurse, Claire releases my hand, gives me a "keep your pecker up", wink.

I follow cuddly blonde Nurse lady through to an Apricot room(meant to make the experience more relaxing), with a chair and examination couch, I am asked to strip to the waist and put on a bat man like cape, I feel a bit of a prat, but do so.

My Consultant, mine in the loosest connotation, but he does make you feel like his only patient ignoring the swelling of patents outside my room. Mr Consultant introduces me to Jean the Breast Care Nurse. We nod a friendly hello. He goes through my Case File and previous notes of Cyst.

The examination of "Bert" is very professional. Both breasts are checked, normal healthy side first to get general map of how tissue felt below, then the other, signs of dimpling, puckering, discharge were looked for and not found, however "Bert" did me proud showing his full figure.

Fluid is Aspirated (Syringe used to draw fluid from my lump). I don't feel a thing, surprisingly. This will now be sent to the lab for tests I am told.

The Nurse smiles at me reassuringly throughout the process.

I can get dressed now.

Once clad, Mr Consultant explains this sample will be sent to the lab, results will be back in three weeks' time. I should make an appointment to return then. I am given a card to tell the receptionist this.

I say "Thank you! "And that I will see him then.

Bald Bird

Claire stands up on seeing me, I'm still, slightly red in the face. Make the afore said appointment, leave the ward, discussing what had happened.

I tell Claire "I wish they could just give me the results now; I would give them every penny I had".

Three weeks is a very long time to wait.

Bald Bird

It's getting bigger

Things calm down during the next couple of days; I carry on working, carry on being a wife and mother.

Mick and I lay in bed one evening; I run my hand over Bert...my stomach lunges. "Mick it's getting bigger!" he laughs, thinking I'm referring to his nether regions. No, my lump, I tell him He feels, agrees, suggests I go back to the GP. My regular GP is unavailable. I see another. This GP offers to try and Aspirate- inserts fine needle, to drain lump, take and use for lab sample, he tries twice to no avail.

I say I think that is enough, the GP's face echoes my realisation. Inform GP I will make appointment with Breast Clinic. Should have gone back there in hindsight. Leave the surgery with inner sense of foreboding.

Mick's home. I tell him. He tells me I should leave the bloody thing alone, remind him that it was upon his insistence that I skedaddled to the GP in panic (not wholly true but that was my take on it at that moment).

Anyway, that night after tucking up the cherubs, my breast begins to throb like hell. Sit quietly, don't tell Mick. Hit the kitchen for Paracetamol. Take these every four hours.

Burn, burns go away; come again another day, its midnight, sleeping beauty snores contentedly by my side. I phone the Emergency Doctors number, as pain is horrendous. Doctor calmly tells me to continue with pain killers; however, I am taking too many he tells me. Asks me if my stomach feels sore, it does, tells me the correct dosage I should now take, advises me to phone the Breast Clinic first thing.

Bald Bird

Today is now Monday, Mr Consultant isn't in Clinic, so make an appointment for tomorrow.

The next day, Claire once again accompanies me to the Clinic. Jean the Breast Nurse calls me into the side room, examines breast, that now holds a lump the size of an entrenched ping pong ball.

I give Jean an update, she gets a colleague Consultant, he advises I attend a Mammogram, for this Thursday, also Mr Consultant will be able to see me after., Jean confirms this.

I dress. tears of fright, tensed up emotion, wave up through me. I ask what the lump could be; the Consultant tells me gently that he wouldn't hazard a guess, not without the lab report and Mammogram.

Tears pour uncontrollably down my face; Jean asks if I'm ok, the Consultant replies, sardonically "obviously not!" Jean offers me a hanky, goes and books appointment with Mr Consultant's secretary, to coincide with Mammogram appointment. I take the card and leave.

I join Claire. "They don't know what it is! I have to wait for the lab report."

Claire diplomatically takes charge, leads me to our office, and gives me hot coffee and chocolate biscuits. I emerge 1 hour later, still a tearful sobbing wreck. Claire had been a star; she has my eternal gratitude.

I reach the car, get in somehow. Phone Mick on my mobile, can't talk for crying,

"Meet you at home," I say.

Bald Bird

Drive home, imagining my funeral, my kids! Nearly ram a shitty coloured Metro up the arse, woman glares through her rear-view mirror, she mouths obscenities.

I give her the two-finger salute, life is too short, and I laugh despite myself.

Make the rest of the journey home safely, fall into husband's arms, gabble out that they don't know what it is. Our Childminder gives me a hug. Diplomatically leaves.

Evening. Mum phones. Be positive she says.

"It's that naughty Cyst again", she wishes I had let her pay for me to go privately, like last time. I say that the treatment I am getting with the NHS is superb, that the time difference would be no different. We carry on discussing her move into the house opposite us, the Holiday House we fondly call it. I clean there on a regular basis during the summer.

Mums house currently being a health risk, due to a cracked, broken drain somewhere in the bowels of her house. Which when sitting in her sitting room, having a cup of tea, is similar to sitting in the public lav. I'm sure you can imagine. Mum will live opposite of us for about two weeks; actually, it turned out to be nearly three months in all. The kids were ecstatic at having "Little Nanny" so close.

We said "goodbyes, I love you". Funny how that has crept in, ending our phone conversations recently.

Mick takes me to the hospital for my Mammogram, etc.

I have now found the loneliest place on the planet, a small cubicle, awaiting the Mammogram machine.

Bald Bird

I wear a cape round my shoulders somewhat like a superhero, just wish I had the Super Chest to go with the image. My boobs get their mug shots, I then go for an Ultrasound, and Mick is invited to join me for support. They pour gel over my breast, just like a Pregnancy Scan. I now see my baby.

The Doctor puts her hand reassuringly on mine. Mr Consultant sees the results.

I'm booked in for a "Lumpectomy" in three days' time. That will be the end of "Bert" I think to myself.

"Hahaha" giggles fate. That's what you think.

My journey and all the people in my life were about to ride an emotional roller coaster, that would cover the next year.

I know where, and what I'll be doing the New Year's Eve for the year 2000, it won't be going to Bristol like Last year.

Bald Bird

Operation Lumpectomy

I pack my bag, nightie, towels, toothbrush, and photo of the children.

Kiss my mum goodbye, and cherubs, smiling and cajoling kids not to tie poor Nanny up for too long, blackmail etc, they laugh wish me good luck and say see you soon.

Anyway, the operation goes well, and after I have the best ever sleep; being total knackered, the nurses teased saying I was like waking the dead. That evening I was asked if I wished to go home, in which I declined, snuggling down in my warm bed. Feeling totally cosseted and spoilt.

On checking my operation scar the next morning find a wider excision than expected, this raises issues in my mind, like why? Nurse says to wait for the results, that will take fifteen days to return. An appointment is made for then. Mick arrives and escorts me home.

Kids go wild on my return; Emily promises they had been gentle with Little Nanny, then runs off giggling with George.

My entire family phone during evening, and friends.

We are shattered, Mick feels horny, so we go to bed and enjoy, carefully, and gently.

Bald Bird

Fifteen days later

We sit in the Breast Clinic. Mick reads a car mag, showing me various car models that take his fancy. I glance and make a derogatory comment about cars being phallic symbols...did he really want a Mini?!

Jean the Breast care Nurse, flits here and there, comes over eventually and gives me a warm hug. My name is called; we go to the Consultation room.

Mr Consultant offers a seat after shaking our hands warmly, I'm slightly embarrassed

As mine is damp and clammy.... again.

Mr Consultant speaks. My heart pounds.

He's sorry to tell me that my so-called Cyst was Cancer: A Malignant Tumour.

It was a Stage 3 Ductal C+ T2 C, 3 NI ER Neg. The tumour had been completely removed, however Mr Consultant felt that the tumour was Margin line, and that for a better result, it would be wise to remove the surrounding tissue. Mr Consultant spoke gently, and kindly. (The above paragraph does not portray his absolute professionalism, which is due to my poor memory, that of being in shock, limits my memory of all the conversation, I would like to stress that I couldn't have been dealt with in a kinder way.)

Mr Consultant explains gently my options- that I can have a larger tissue area removed, or that a Mastectomy followed by immediate reconstruction was also an option.

Bald Bird

Also explained was that for them to fully diagnose me, Lymph nodes would be removed and sampled (tested), depending on how many nodes were affected would help plan further treatment. Such as Chemotherapy.

First, I want to know what a Stage three meant.

"If it were a dog, I ask, what breed would it be?"

"A Rottweiler, but although it is an aggressive Cancer, we have caught it early. When we have the results of your Lymph nodes that will give us the full picture.

I say that I would rather have a Mastectomy, have it all taken away, my inner thoughts thinking that this would give less chance of re occurrence. I realise that I have already chosen before I had even walked through the door.

Mr Consultant draws diagrams of different reconstruction techniques. I opt for the back Dorsal Muscle (the back muscle is brought round to the chest with its own blood supply and forms part of the breast) and Silicone implant. Later I have the option of a Nipple Tattoo.

"Please take a few days to think about it. When we meet again, we can arrange the surgery date. I have free the 15th and the 22nd of December", Mr Consultant looks at me to gauge which date suits.

I say the 15th.

"Well let's meet in two days, and book." Mr Consultant stands as we say goodbye.

Bald Bird

Jean gestures us to follow her, we go to her little room, and all others are occupied. I picture women wailing and crying, throwing themselves on the floor in despair.

I think I have been given a death sentence at this point, I actually haven't but that is how I felt just at that moment. Jean asks us to sit.

We do. I cry. Tears of sheer fear course down my face. Mick is also in tears; Jean gives us space. She then talks to us. Explaining the diagnosis, and that all was not doom or gloom. I was young and would recover quickly from the surgery. Jean thought I had made a good choice for surgery, and that she too would have taken that path.

Jean hands us leaflets that we can read later, about Breast cancer Diagnosis, in the back pages Support Addresses and phone numbers. Mastectomy information on Silicone

Breast Surgery, how safe Silicone is etc.

I am shaking, and feel that I'm now losing my grip, I tell Jean all my bottled-up feelings and fears, I can't sleep, I can't eat, I'm so scared. Jean suggests that I visit my GP, just for a short-term measure, get some Anti-depressants, just to take the pressure off a bit. (I do this, and it definitely got me through). I arrange an appointment time with Jean to see Mr Consultant for two days' time.

Two days later the date for surgery is set for the 22nd December 1999, and I do still go for the Mastectomy.

I never in the world dreamed that my wish for the Millennium would be that I would live. I vowed that no lump (you Bert), would rob me of my life, I loved my life, my family, and besides we had a party to attend New Year's Eve, and we would be going! That I promised myself.

Bald Bird

Breaking the bad news

You know, sometimes the hardest thing in life is telling the ones you love bad news. I was dreading it.

Having got the results of my Lumpectomy, left me in no doubt that I had a fight on my hands, a Mastectomy and then the possibility of Chemotherapy afterwards.

Mum opened the door, and just by looking at my face knew all in the garden wasn't rosy. She bundled me in the door, and held me close, once seated on the settee, through wrenching sobs told her the results. Mum in her wisdom told me we weren't beat yet, and that things, were luckily, so luckily at the treatable stage, we had a chance. Emotionally I'm shagged, knackered, my brain hurts. Everything hurts.

The thought of dying, not seeing my children as adults hurts, my husband of only a few months remarrying some full busted blonde hurts, running off with my Life Insurance hurts (he wouldn't, but you begin to think like this), being forgotten and replaced hurts.

Mick phones his parents with the results, Kathleen from next door pops in, to see how things went, I tell her, through sips of Whisky (a small plus in this situation).

"Oh dear!" Kath looks weepy.

Mick tells her things aren't bad; we're being positive, he tells her. He thinks I don't notice the look he gives her. Our mates from over the road, (number 24, we're 27) come in, we all sit together, and I get hugged a lot. People glancing through the window probably think we're having a wife swapping party!

Bald Bird

Eventually people leave. Emily my daughter comes in complaining of hunger pangs, we all laugh. Thank god for children, whatever's going on they keep normality.

Feed kids, and then chat about my decision on having Mastectomy, followed by immediate reconstruction. Mum says not to bother with the reconstruction as this a large operation in its own right. I say I'm only 32, I love the beach, and want to get back to normal as quickly as possible. I understand where mum was coming from, but I'm being offered a gift here, reconstruction surgery has quite a long waiting list, plus when I had come round from surgery not that much would be different.

Two days later I confirm this with Mr Consultant, he clearly explains the surgical procedure; he draws diagrams, explaining the use of my back muscle to be brought round to my chest, plus silicone implant. Ten days in hospital.

My mum has decided to take off work, to be my and my children's carer, I tell Mr Consultant. Surgery is set for 22.12.99 over the Christmas period; it hits me that this is not what I planned for the Millennium.

I have a party to go to, maybe god willing I could still make it, I'd hate for us to miss Steve and Sharon's party, there parties were legendary.

Ten days before the operation date, I pop into Dorchester Hospital to give medical background etc.

Everyone mentally prepares for the upcoming date of the Op. Mick returns to Bristol every other weekend, maintaining contact with the girls. I see that he feels

Bald Bird

guilty at leaving us, me. I encourage him to go but miss him so much.

Me and the kids carry on going to mums across the road for healthy meals, and

Scrummy teas, long walks. Life carries on.

I phone Natalie; Monday am (my boss) and tell her the results.

Natalie then phones her manager. This is extremely helpful, takes a load off my shoulders, as don't think I could get through the whole explanation without bursting into tears. Claire phones me that evening, giving me love from everyone at work. I receive cards from them in the following days.

I find that emotionally I'm really struggling, feel really down. I visit my GP again, who suggests a short course of Antidepressants, just to see me through the next few weeks, month or so. I agree.

The next few weeks drags by. Antidepressants kick in, which make me feel a bit spacey, removed from reality. Without the tablets I become very down. I believe that my diagnosis can only lead to one outcome, cheerful or what?

All I can think about is "Cancer". I read all leaflets concerning this subject, front and back, I even have a secret stash in the bathroom, in case I need a quick top up of knowledge, my family pretend they don't know about my secret hoard. They watch sadly at my obsessive behaviour.

The Millennium is fast approaching, we wrap Christmas pressies, put up the decorations. Emily and George bicker, I burst into tears. I don't want my children arguing on what could be my last Christmas.

Bald Bird

I carry on going to work; we have the Christmas lunch combined Becky's leaving bash, the hospital canteen is transformed to a sparkling grotto. We toast Becky, wish her all the best in her new life in Australia complete with Doctor Boyfriend Matt.

I will miss her; we have become close. I wonder as I hug my colleagues wishing Merry Christmas, when will I return?" Happy Christmas, cracking New Year everyone!

Becky and I leave together, in the car park give each other a big hug, a skinny builder walks by puffing on a rolly, gives us a "raving lesbians", glare. We both laugh and go our separate ways.

At home we celebrate Christmas one week early, due to the fact I will be ensconced in a hospital bed on the real day. We hug, kiss and thank for our wonderful pressies, my chest holds in the hot anger that I feel a this very moment, fear, jealousy, that if I might not be here for the next Christmas how long would it be before another woman takes my place in their hearts, of those I love. Irrational fear, but that is what I think.

That weekend we go to Mick's parents (Norma and Sid) with Emily and George.

We have a wonderful pre-Christmas again! Mick's girls are also with us. We open pressies, have a great Christmas dinner, and lazy after noon, snowflakes start to fall, and thicken. As we look out later the snow has settled so we all tog up and go for a walk. The local playing field looks beautiful with the freshly laid snow; we all do snow angels and build a snow man.

A wonderful weekend, all too soon it's time to go home.

Bald Bird

Dear Diary 22.12.99

I pack once again. Mum looks after the children, on my leaving gives me a big hug. The kids believe this to be the beginning of a rugby scrum, and pile on in.

Extricate myself, Mick and I bolt for the car, we listen to the Mavericks at full volume. Ironically stopping at the local garage for a pack of fags for Mick.

Arrive, check in, named, and numbered in the form of a wrist band. I Am given a rather swish electrical bed that apparently could get into all sorts of positions.

Mr Consultant arrives, greeting me warmly, then asks me to undo my garments (curtains are drawn) draws with black marker intended surgical arrears. Once happy with this, says I can get dressed again now. Asks if I have any concerns, surgical or otherwise. I ask him to just check under my armpit, I think I'm getting a swelling there (Paranoid) ...all is fine.

(Have you ever become obsessive, you know like that disorder where you keep checking if you've left the gas on, or having got into bed, think did I lock the door? Well you bloody well know you have locked the door, but you still haul yourself out of that lovely warm bed, go down the cold stairs, and check. Well, every nodule, tiny lump or bump that lies under my skin gets checked and checked again. I find new lumps that definitely weren't there yesterday were they?!?)

Australian Anaesthetist arrives, explains he will be monitoring me during op, and post-operative for pain control. Will be managed

Bald Bird

by Morphine injections. Great I say, there is an upside to all this! We both laugh. He leaves.

The Florist arrives at the same time as Karyn (S.A.L.T), Karyn leaves a Christmas Cacti and card at reception as doesn't want to disturb me. The florist bares a bunch of the most beautiful white roses, courtesy of my man. I hug Mick. Mick is asked not to stay too long to let me get settled in, we have a huge cuddle, I'm frightened I cry, I put my head down, squeeze him and ask him to go. Mick tells me he will stay in Dorchester town centre all day; he will come back when I come out of theatre.

I will now use a diary to track my wandering thoughts, will write when next able.

Bald Bird

Dear Diary 23.12.99

I'm in an electrical bed. I can hear the rain beating on the windows. Have a looked at my scars, two symmetrical, blue stitches like fishing nylon hold me together, and a neat clean, mound has replaced my breast, and I feel bruised.

I have no nipple. My armpit is numb. But I'm alive!! Tubes drain my back, and my newly constructed breast. I remember now being wheeled to theatre. I fall asleep.

I remember waking in the night, shouting, Morphine is injected, I sleep again.

Breakfast, painkillers, Nurses give me a bed bath, what angels! I didn't feel humiliated as I thought I might, just mildly self-conscious. Now sitting on the commode was a different thing! But needs must. I feel weak and wobbly.

Visitors pop in to see me, Anne from the Children's Centre, Also Jill.

Mick comes in soaked; he tells me that our central heating has packed in at home, we guess at the odds of resurrecting a plumber on Christmas Eve, Mick rushes off, forever the optimist for the hunt. God, he looks knackered

Claire pokes her head round the door we have a laugh together, she goes. Mum and kids arrive mid-afternoon...I fall asleep, unaware that the day has blended into night. I wake up alone.

Dear God, if you can hear me, I promise that from now on I will lead an exemplarity life, if only you will let me live to see my children grown, please I will give back tenfold, please......I fall asleep.

Bald Bird

Crappy night's sleep, full of nightmares. Dream a blackbird is flying at me, gets caught in my hair.... I can't pull it out. Wake up bolt upright, screaming, or so I think. A Nurse injects me in the thigh, sleep, peaceful full heavy sleep.

Bald Bird

Dear Diary 24.12.99

Christmas eve! 8.00am.

I have a visitor, Mr Consultants Surgeon assistant, plus a nurse. Show him new boob. He examines drains; three tubes that come from wounds: two in front one behind. I think I must look like an Octopus. All are working well; I wish I could have a bath, feel sweaty, tired, and grumpy. However, wish the staff a Merry Christmas, and could they think Mr Consultant for my wonderfully constructed new boob. They say they will.

In the midst of this conversation two lovely bouquets and a large teddy with a balloon attached appears around the curtain, this is from Mick's cousin and family, from Merseyside.

Emotion suddenly hits me; from all the weeks before seeming to burst out of me. I cry.

I have a new friend!, the cleaner, I am the only patient on the ward, all other patients have been discharged, we chat about this and that she then carries on with her multitudes of duties before her, with a cheery goodbye she continues forth. The nurses are lovely and join me on their tea breaks.

Claire pops in and goes. I wonder in my mind has the Cancer gone, has the cancer gone. **Bert, do you miss me, I sure as hell don't miss you.**

Mick comes in frozen to bits. We have a long cuddle.

Bald Bird

Dear Diary 25.12.99

Christmas Day, I have had a bath! Oh bliss.

Go with new roommate, who came in the middle of the night (Suspected heart attack) to Holy Communion. Meet the Vicar who I regularly see in passing on Hardy Ward where I work, he smiles a hello. Jane from occupational Therapy is playing the piano. Now it feels like Christmas -sings Amazing Grace, I feel like I've been given mine.

Waiting for me are Mick, Ems, and George, they look shattered, open pressies.

From George a candle with silver stars.

Ems a gorgeous angel in a beautiful card. Children are restless, uncomfortable in their surroundings, ask Mick to take them home, I feel really pissed off as really want them to stay longer. Now I feel sorry for myself, down. Mick tells me: chin up. I feel like telling him to piss off. It's not him lying in this sodding bed is it? He can go out into the fresh air and escape. I can't. Then I feel guilty. He's looking after my children, working and is worried sick. God I'm a selfish cow. Selfish cow snuggles down and goes to sleep. I sleep. I wake and my mum is with me, I'm so pleased to see her it hurts.

Bald Bird

Dear Diary 26.12.99

Excellent night's sleep. Felt low yesterday. The ward nurses invite me into the staff room for mince pies, and coffee, bless 'em. Things like that make such a difference. I then get shown a side room, that has a TV and a bed in.

I can use that if I want to.

9.00am.Ward round. Bare all. Dr agrees one drain clear; this can now be taken out.

Oh, what joy, hope it doesn't hurt too much I'm such a coward where pain is concerned.

I'm given a Paracetamol, (I know this is a Placebo effect!) in preparation for drain removal. Mick is here phew! Hand holder, gas and air on offer.

Half an hour later, inside ward I lay down, quivering slightly. "Deep breaths" says the nurse, I do, and the strangest sensation follows as the plastic tube slides from under my skin and back muscle, out of my body. Wow! I feel slightly dizzy, and scuttle off back to my ward as soon as the procedure is done

Two tubes to go before freedom. Mick and I go to the TV room, other patients and guests turn and look at me. I carry the bulbs that the tubes drain into in a material handbag. I hope they think I've got my knitting needles in there. I say a bubbly hello.

They seem to all relax.

Bald Bird

Dear Diary 27.12.99

Good night's sleep. My heart does beating somersaults as my Grandparents, Aunty Steff and my mum also walk through after them. Never underestimate the power of good that a family visit does.

Chat for an hour, then I'm suddenly very tired. Mum sees this, and whisks everyone home. Hugs all round first though.

I feel restless now everyone's gone and can't settle even though I am tired. I get up slowly and cautiously minding my tubes, pick up my drain bags and wander down the ward...and come across leaflets by the ward door. The leaflets are on Breast cancer.

Feel depressed, on my beating this Bastard disease. Stand and talk to the passing nurses. To bed now, do really feel physically tired. Write diary first.

Night. Night. Write again tomorrow.

3.00am.

Get woken up by an elderly lady being brought in, lady in her 60s.Comes in to have her abdomen drained. Ovarian Cancer she tells me positively. She's just come back from seeing her daughter in Australia. Sleep.

Ward round.

Drs Says I can now have other drains out. Have first drain out, this is draining my front, my reconstructed breast, it slides out easily, the second pulls a bit, but all is fine.

Guess what the Dr then tells me......! YEP I CAN BLOODY WELL GO HOME, I CAN GO HOME, ICAN GO HOME, HOME, HOME, HOME! BLOODY HELL HOME!

Bald Bird

Mum pops in with Gran and Grandad, and Steff, looks thoroughly worried when I tell her I can go home. Mum worries that I'm not worried, I get cross and tell her I'm so ready to go, mum still feels it's too early.

Looking back of course, I now see the overwhelming responsibility that mum must have felt, worried that she might not be able to cope with looking after me and my whole household. My Grandparents have rented the holiday house in my street, they say they will help.

Doctor comes round, explains follow up treatment, possibility of Chemo, stitches out after tenth day, that will be New Year's Day then, The Millennium, and the year 2000!

Please I say, one day won't make any difference, could we do it for a day after, he laughs following my drift. 02.01.2000 is agreed upon for stitch removal. I can go home tomorrow. Mick pops in 8.30pmish, I tell him I can go home tomorrow, to celebrate we go for a walk around the hospital, we look at my photo with the other staff members celebrating the opening of the new wing. Mick points to Claire's photo and says she's gorgeous. There's me just had my tit off and he's ogling someone else, a word to the wise this really isn't a good move. I storm off. Mick runs after me; I can certainly shift when I'm pissed off. Mick says he didn't mean it like that, being female I store this for back up material, but forgive him, just about.

Bald Bird

D-Day 28.12.99 I'm going home!

Go home today. Crappy night's sleep last night, late night admission of a lady wearing an oxygen mask...poor love rattled and wheezed all night.

12.15pm Surprise visitors for me! Norma and Sid Mick's parents arrive. I am having my lunch they say they'll come back in an hour. They are helping Mick with some house renovations, Norma has done our ironing...apparently, we nearly have central heating now. Norma and Sid leave after an hour, I sit and chat with other patient's relatives, one of the nurses brings in her new fella, we laugh, and he goes shy.

Teatime Mick at last arrives to take me home, I've been packed since 10.00am this morning. We give my flowers to remaining patients, and fresh flowers and card to nurses. This seems such a small gesture for all the hard work and dedication they put into their work.

Feel like I've been let out of prison, fresh cold air hits me, I feel rather shaky on the old pins. Luckily, Mick has parked close, wheelchair not needed. I sit through the journey home, feeling relieved that part of my treatment is over. I can't wait to see Ems and George. I will make that New Year Party after all!

Arrive home, to squeals of joy from my babies, we hug in the hallway, eventually they let me go, I go through the hallway upstairs.

I feel disorientated slightly, put things in bedroom. Mum has brought a whole new fresh white cotton linen set for our bed. It is gorgeous. I feel tears in my eyes but push them back. Mum comes over from across the street, gives me a gentle hug trying

Bald Bird

not to squash my rebuild, Gran and Granddad also, with Aunty Steff.

Jesus I've missed my kids.

Once I'm settled my visiting family say they're off but will be back again in the morning.

Go to bed early; find it difficult to get comfy, now I'm not in my super-duper electric bed. I wriggle and huff and puff, then hubby makes me a triangle out of my pillows. He nods off, I stare at the ceiling.

Bald Bird

Dear Diary 29.12.99

Where my back muscle used to be (Now part of my breast) fluid begins to fill. This is really uncomfortable. Go to hospital. Jean Breast care Nurse drains with a syringe.   Ah bliss comfortable once more.

At home watching television I'm suddenly aware that every programme has women with bulging breasts. Nipples jutting out, juggling in my face, taunting me. I storm off to bed. Mick follows.

I grizzle pathetically. I'm not feminine anymore. I'm not who you married, I've lost my sexual appeal, confidence in my appearance. Mick dives off downstairs and brings back with him our wedding photograph. Mick tells me I am the same woman in that photo, I have not changed in his eyes.... I try and understand what he's saying.

But you see, lying in this bed is a totally different person, physically, mentally, and spiritually.... totally to that woman in the wedding photo that Mick is looking into the eyes of.

Mick spookily reads my thoughts and cuddles me gently. "We'll get through this, us, the kids, I love you." He kisses my forehead and then gets up to re hang our photo in the living room downstairs.

Perhaps I think change can be a good thing, it has certainly made me reassess our life. I lay still, thinking of all the good things I have in my life. You know, all the things you take for granted: a house, healthy children, a loving family and husband. Mick switches off the bedroom light, snuggles up to me, and slowly as the sky begins to get light, drift off to sleep.

44

Bald Bird

I have decided not to write my diary daily now, as want to get on with daily living, just get on with family life. Mick collects his mum's triangle pillow on his next visit to Bristol.

Sleep comes much easier with this aid.

Bald Bird

Results of Lymph nodes

Mick and I get ready, be still oh beating heart -my appointment to get my results is nearer this time, Weymouth hospital. We drive and arrive twenty minutes later. There is no problem parking at this hospital. I know this hospital well, as I covered the outpatients for Speech Therapy, with Claire. I lead Mick through reception and to the waiting area and sit waiting for my name to be called.

As if on cue, another Speechie (slang for Speech Therapist) walks down the corridor towards us. We say hi, how are you, all the time my eye is trained on the room which holds the answers to the next few years of my life...hopefully. She picks this up wishing me good luck, calls her patient and they follow her back to her Therapy room.

My name is eventually called, not that the waiting time has been long, just seems that way. Dr D introduces herself, she is an Oncologist, she in other words checks blood of Cancer patients. "Have I had my results yet?", "No" I say.

She tells me that I have had 19 Lymph nodes removed, a minimal amount of Cancer was found in 1. The whole tumour was removed successfully, however Chemotherapy would be necessary. FEC (I'm not swearing, that is the name of the Chemo treatment.) 6 cycles.

Or in other words, 6 sessions in layman's terms.

Dr D then introduced us to another Breast care Nurse and leaves us to chat about follow up treatment.

I talk through my results, were they good, would I be ok?

Bald Bird

The nurse says the results were good, but she couldn't give me an outcome. I'm given leaflets, and a form to claim for the cost of an NHS wig. This done, we drive off to Poole,

We find the wig shop.

Wig hunting can be hilarious, Mick tries on a curly short haired platinum blonde wig that looks so funny against his swarthy Italian looks, he resembles a rather confused Rod Stewart, he swings in the chair grinning profanely, and he makes me and the Shop Assistant roar with laughter.

I purchase a wig called "Linda", it is a red, sandy, colour, straight, and shoulder length. I sign the form, hand over my voucher, and then still wearing the wig, we exit the shop. We are going to watch other people to see if they notice it's a wig or not!

I feel like a special agent undercover, as we slip down the street and into the local supermarket, I'm scared the wig will slip, it feels hot and itchy, and I feel like I have a sign above my head. Stating-

"Bald Bird wearing a wig." I'm suddenly tired and need a drink.

We go hit a local café, once we have got coffee and cake, we find a quiet corner. Mick squeezes my leg under the table, he tells me I'm a hot babe...ahhh.

"Does it look real though?" I pursue. "Yeah, you look drop dead gorgeous!" Mick not realizing what he has said, smiles, bless him, my silver-tongued Cavalier. We go home.

Jean the Breast care Nurse phones, I give her my results, she says that's a fantastic result couldn't be better. Arrange to meet

Bald Bird

Jean downstairs of the hospital on the 1st February to look round Chemo ward.

Show kids my wig, having removed it before pulling up home. George thrusts it on his head, we roar with laughter, he looks just like his sister! We go to the holiday house for a coffee and to show George off in his wig.

Bald Bird

Next Step

Today I go with mum, to see Jean the Breast care nurse; she gives me a warm hug. Mum asks various questions about the up and coming Chemo, and what should we expect.

Jean gives information on how the body reacts, how over the sessions one's immune system becomes weaker, so a wise move is to stay away from fluey people, or coughs and colds etc.

Jean then leads us to the Chemo ward; we take things slowly as I tend to get breathless.

We stop momentarily for me to gather second wind; I am then introduced to the nurses.

The room once again is a pretty peach colour, with rows of comfy seats, just like any other waiting room, I don't know what I was expecting. We say goodbye to Jean and thank her for showing me around.

Mum drives us home. Thank you mum you're a star. Xxx

Bald Bird

The Millennium! 2000!

Happy New Year One and all!

It is sufficient to say we all made the party. Mick, myself, Ems and George, our next-door neighbours, all wander up the street together.

I felt very light and fragile.

Mick told me I looked beautiful in my long black and white dress. I had looked at my reflection, it is not the real me that stares back, I look into the hollow-eyed thin person. But shrug and think what the hell. Emily came up to bring me downstairs.

We go to the party.

I wonder if you can remember what you did for the Millennium. I know I will never forget.

Happy New Year Everyone.

Joie de vivre!

Bald Bird

First Chemo Session

Mick comes with me. The nurse explains the procedure as I settle myself into a comfy chair where the Chemo is administrated. They will put a needle into a vein that will be linked to the Chemotherapy treatment. FEC.

The drug is made up of three types of drug each one will give a separate sensation.

1. I may feel the sensation of ants marching across my chest, forehead, and nasal area.

2. I may feel lightheaded, well I've always been rather scatty...so!

3. Metallic taste in mouth.

Whilst this is being explained to me, I take in the other ladies, some are wearing wigs, some aren't, some wear cold caps (Supposed to stop your hair loss) they seem to be all at different stages of treatment. One lady is being told that she can't have her final course of Chemo today as her blood count is too low. She is really pissed off, but takes it on the chin, and re-appoints.

"How long does it take for the hair loss to start?" I ask. I am told roughly about two sessions. My friend Liz is getting married in two months, I wonder if I'll have hair...the answer to that is I wore Linda that day.

I recognize a lady from the day of my positive diagnosis, she has waist long straight blonde hair, and her name is Jean. Before we start our first session, we swap phone numbers, book times to

Bald Bird

attend our second session together. We become allies from thence forth.

Mick leaves me with Jean and will return an hour later. Jean and I sit, get lined up and chat. We take each other's mind off what we're doing. The treatment surges through our veins.

I do feel the ants crossing my forehead and chest. Mick arrives just as the Chemo finishes. I say goodbye to everyone. Say see you next time.

Mick drives me home; I feel like crap and promptly burst into tears on Ridgeway hill. Mick carries on driving me home.

It just isn't bloody fair, what have I done to deserve this.

During that first week, I drink lots of water. Mum has brought me a water filter jug that is by the side of my bed. It is constantly refilled, as I drink to flush out the toxins,

I am wiped out, no energy, and sleepy. I spend hours drifting in and out of sleep. Below our bedroom drones the daily hubbub of life, mum cooks, washes, irons. I feel left out, and useless.

Through the constant care, and the fabulous cooking skills of mum, I rally daily, each day feeling a little stronger. I must be feeling better, I think to myself as daytime TV is boring me rigid.

I lay in bed dreaming; Kilroy is coming on with Special Birthday ideas. Ummm I think raising my head, Mick's birthday was coming up, and I wanted to do something unusual.

Kilroy announced: "Balloon rides, Helicopter rides, and Racing days."

That was it! Mick adored The Grand Prix; I would arrange a Race Day!

Bald Bird

Our next-door neighbour, a work colleague of Mick's had done a Race Day, I would pop round and get the address and info when back on my feet. Feeling Smug, I curl over and guess what, promptly throw up.

The next day, feeling better, I dress and pop round next door and pick up the address for Race Days. The place is a bit too far out for us, so I wait for our house to clear and phone Mick's mother.

Norma tells me there is a place called "Castle Combe Circuit" about 15 minutes away from them. We could all go up and stay with them. It would be a good break for all of us.

I phone Castle Combe Circuit, and book. I wanted Mick's birthday, but this was fully booked, they would send me the booking vouchers, that way Mick could choose a date that would work. The brochures arrive a few days later, Ems brings me the letter, we sit cuddled up in bed and read. They offer 4x4 drives, skid pan days, Racing Days. Ems and I think the Racing Day is perfect. Ems passes me the phone; I read them my credit card details. Ems and I hug we're so excited.

I can now relax.

George and Emily love to cook, so when he comes home from school, we set about making Mick's birthday cake, we have a laugh measuring, mixing, and making a general mess. George and Ems divide the empty bowl to lick out the bowl after; we look at our work of art, which resembles a Frisbee. Well it's the thought that counts.

Bald Bird

Mick's Birthday - 05.02.00

The first chinks of light appear through our curtains, it's so quiet, I can hear hushed whispering the rustle of paper, then a slight punch up begins in the hall; I have to laugh at my little treasures they try so hard. I count to myself, 10, 9, 8,7....

"Happy birthday Mick!" in bounds a leaping gazelle in the shape of my daughter, closely followed by a crumpled George. Their arms are laden with little pressies, all at various stages of presentation. Arguments ensue, of what pressies should be opened first. Emily wins.

Mick isn't yet fully awake; his hair is looking punk-rocker-ish. He bears the resemblance of a rabbit caught in the headlights. Eventually it dawns on him, his birthday has arrived. "Thanks Ems, deodorant." George and Ems pass the next present between them-a clue to the up and coming scenario.

Mick whoops, "It's a toy Formula 1 Racing Car", and kisses both Ems and George, Ems grins, George scowls pretending he didn't enjoy the attention, but did really. A silly boy grin covers Mick's face. Between you and me I think he has twigged.

"Now my pressie!" I hand him the gold envelope. Mick opens. I think he's going to burst; the kids roll around the bed laughing, Mick nearly goes to leap out of the bed, I restrain, reminding him of his natural state. He punches the air instead. Once initial excitement has subsided go through possible dates for him to book. Norma and Sid phone to wish a Happy Birthday.

George dashes off downstairs returning with the cooked Frisbee, and we all munch on slices of chocolate cake for breakfast.

Happy days.

Bald Bird

2nd Chemo

Okay. Now my hair has started to fall out. As agreed, Mick that evening gets out the hair clippers. I am given a number 2 crew cut; I have chosen this action, as hair falling out is distressing, so quick restyle is my solution. I now wear a woolly hat to cover the fact that I'm now "A bald Bird!"

My Chemo appointment.

Joan fellow patient is already there, we look at each other and nod...you too, and we are now crew cut twins. We go for our Chemo; our respective other halves leave the ward together.

Dr D checks my blood, to make sure I'm not anaemic or any other thing to cause stop of treatment, all is fine. I get my drugs...ants crawl up my nose and across my forehead.

I'm on a promise today, after treatment we are going to McDonald's for lunch. This is a hit, and always from now on a stop we make. I tell Mick I'm going straight to bed this time, as trying to stay up doesn't pay dividends. I crash.

Mary Poppins alias mum works her miracles in the kitchen. I get up and join my family for tea. I work (I don't have an appetite at present) through the wonderfully nutritious meal before me, I drink gallons of water. I try and make light conversation with all around me.

Then I have an almighty urge...... being toiletry for a minute have to dash to the loo for a number 2. I haven't been for what seems like an eternity...ah bliss I never thought I would so enjoy a poo. Exhausted from the excitement I go to bed. (Get wonderful stuff from Doctors later that week: Lactulose, a blessing for the bound.)

Bald Bird

Downstairs mum continues cooking, singing her God Songs at high decibels, she makes me chuckle as I lay in bed, she warbles away merrily to herself and Ems and George are a captive audience. I doze off. Next thing I know it is dark. The house is quiet, my husband lays cuddled up to me. Mother of the washing, ironing, and comforter of children has gone to her own bed across the way. God Bless you mum, how would I ever manage without you. Thank you for all your hard work and never doubting spirit that supports mine when I'm doubting.

The following day, Mick goes to Bristol to see his girls. This gives me some alone time with my babies. We share this time with mum and go over to the holiday house. We go for a short walk, and then have tea. Play board games and chill.

Mick returns Sunday night; I nag and moan. "What if I dint make it? Scenarios." He is patience itself going through my prognosis. We go to bed mentally shattered.

In the morning I think I've found a lump in my right breast, phone Jean Breast care Nurse, she will check it for me after I've had my third Chemo-here I go again checking, checking...

Bald Bird

Emily and George

Throughout my diagnosis I have tried to be as honest as I could be without trying to frighten Ems and George too much. Emily has a firmer understanding of what we're going through and, bless her, has taken looking after her brother to heart.

It's difficult to keep normality going when such things as illness raises its head within a family, but I think it's important to keep a balance.

Both Ems and George continue to go to school. However, I did phone both schools and inform them of my treatment and asked them to contact me if either child was finding it difficult to cope or was very upset.

Children can be strong, and some cruel. George came home with a bruised face one day, I got out of him gently that a lad had teased him about me having no hair, so George retaliated. They had a punch up in the school yard.

I went to the school the next day and waited for said boy, after school. Drawing him aside warned the little shit never to touch George or tease him again. I was so sodding angry; I think he saw that. Needless to say, this never happened again, as far as I'm aware.

Bald Bird

Something to look forward to!

Mum takes the kids swimming. Mum has membership to a hotel, where there's a pool, with lots of rubber tubes floats, and toys.

Ems and George have hours of fun chasing Little Nanny as they call her around the pool, having play fights with the foam tubes. When they return, frazzled but content Mick suggests as we sit having a tea, juice, he was thinking of doing a loft conversion.

 Emily is thrilled, stairs to get away from George! George could have Emily's room. The planning begins in earnest. Mick draws the plans with Emily and George. I sit back and smile. Something for them to look forward to.

George asks if he can choose the colour for his room, he currently has red and orange his two favourite colours adorning his walls, "sure!" says Mick pulling a face at me," As long as it's not black Georgie!"

 George grins "Well it is my room...!"I know George is joking, hopefully.

The next day work begins on the loft. Mick needs this something to work on, Ems and George need something to look forward to: A future.

Bald Bird

3rd Chemo, 15.03.00

Mum again drives me to Chemo. See Jean about lump in right breast, she believes it to be hormonal. However, appointment is made for a mammogram this Thursday. Dr D has also examined me and agrees this. I have Chemo, Joan my Breast friend joins me, we both look like Army Recruits. Session finishes. Book next session. Mum drives me home. However, we are low on food, so we decide to stop off at Asda to stock up. I am wearing a green woolly hat today, couldn't be arsed with" Linda".

You know, I must be accepting my illness and prepared myself in some way for what would happen next. I was wandering round the veg aisle looking at food I didn't really want to eat, and then wham.

"Hi Kaye, how are you?!" Sean says. Sean is the husband of Karen. Karen and I had our first-born children at the same hospital ward. We became firm friends, and found we lived in the same street. Eventually I moved away from Dorchester to Portland, so we now just bump into each other as and when. But it's always such a treat to see them. Anyway, he carries on teasing me" Smart hat!" I take a deep breath, and say, "Haven't you heard?"! I then calmly explain what has happened to me, about Chemo.

He's great, and asks me questions, am I ok, is there anything I need, he says he's sorry to hear that, me too I say. Sean gives me a big hug. I send my love to his wife, we say goodbye. Just an average conversation in a shopping Isle. Mum rests her hand on my shoulder, gently smiles, puts her arm round my shoulder and leads me on to finish shopping.

Bald Bird

Once home I crash again, I'm knackered. Mum once again over the next five days, cooks, cares, loves. I'm knackered, and look it, my skin looks grey, I am hollow eyed, and I feel and look like a walking skeleton. I have lost lots of weight. I'm feeling low too.

Mick's mum offers us a lifeline and invites us up to Bristol. This means my mum gets a rest, Ems and George have a change of scene. The following weekend we go to Bristol. Feel a bit sick on the journey up, but however we get there.

I am wearing "Linda" and feel a total prat. Mick's parents are kind, and say I look great. Ummmm….   Kitty sits on my knee once we've all settled and starts to pull at my hair, it slides over, and I quickly read just, she pulls and so on the game continues, until Norma calls Kitty off. I'm now feeling very tearful & vulnerable, so slope off upstairs with Ems and George. George is on his Game boy we share. I mutter angrily to myself.

Lunch. I'm not hungry but make the effort.

Cadburys World- our next choice to visit this afternoon, we have a great day, and funny enough chocolate doesn't make me feel sick, now there's a thing!

That night Emily is sick. (Too much choccy.)

Emily asks to stay with Norma and Sid, as still isn't feeling completely pucker when we talk about going swimming. Kitty and Sally really want to go, so does George. Making sure that Emily is settled, happy before we set off. I don't swim, I watch, can't risk getting a bug, or cold just now. On our return Ems is running around the garden and seems much better.

Bald Bird

That evening George gets raging earache, and a temperature of 102, he sleeps in with me and Mick. Were all worn out. In the morning Mick gets Calpol. George rallies later that evening, so we decide to take a slow drive home. It is a few days after that poor Georgie feels well enough to return to school.

See George off to school and decide that I will go into Weymouth. I will go to the Library and get a good book to read. I park the car and walk through the town. I go to the library.

I find an awe-inspiring book, though deeply sad, of a young woman who had Breast cancer. Her name was "Ruth Picardie" the title was "Before I say Goodbye", I can only read a few chapters before tears are pouring down my face. This is a strange need in me, to find out how women my age cope or try to cope with this illness. Ruth did it with courage, that's what I need to know.

Just at that moment I have a terrible feeling, I don't think or can't remember getting a parking ticket... Shit. My memory (Chemo Brain) is really something at the moment. I leave the library bookless, tearstained, and in a panic.

I tank it past the Art Shop, as I do so I see a painting by numbers (Mick is on at me to get a new hobby) a picture of a Norfolk scene, the setting looks just like Burnham Overy Creek, which is where I was born, I have to have it, scrabble in my purse for the change (£1.99 sheer bargain). I steam in- pay in seconds to a rather bemused gentleman, then leg it to the car park.

Grabbing breath, I puff and pant to the car park. Almost unable to bare to look, to see if I did indeed get a parking ticket. Peer through one eye at my car window screen. I hadn't bought a

Bald Bird

ticket (Crap). Even more surprising (I now firmly believe I have a Guardian Angel) was I don't Have a yellow plastic wallet containing a car park fine!

Life is great!

Bald Bird

Paranoid Thursday

I wait patiently at the Breast clinic. I have become acclimatised to this clinic now and feel strangely reassured just being here.

I'm now in the Peachy room, having been called through for my check up, wearing the cape of Decency. Mr Consultant enters the room. Mr Consultant checks my healthy side, for the lump. But bless it, it has decided to do a hiding act, or hormonally disappeared. I go red and feel like a pillock.

I have the ultrasound, this shows nothing.

I dress and leave and drive home.

I recognize that an irrational fear has got hold of me. I think I need to talk this trough with a professional, I keep thinking cancer is springing up inside my internal organs like mushrooms.

I phone my GP when I get in, who refers me onto a Counsellor:

Someone I can really talk to; someone I don't have to be brave in front of. Someone I can be honest and say how truly frightened I am.

Bald Bird

Counselling Session

I now face a situation I'm uncomfortable with. But recognize I need support.

I'm going for my Counselling session. Now this is cute because I have done some training in Counselling, but now have the tables turned and I'm on the receiving end.

I change clothes about eight times before I eventually get I my car, put on the stereo

Fairly loud to cover my beating heart.

Once I arrive at my destination car park I slowly pull in and park up, truthfully I   consider doing a quick u-turn going back out again, how wet am I. Decide to pull myself together and pull on my fetching blue floppy hat. Get out of the car assertively as possible and flop through the door up to the receptionist.

Give my name to Mrs Smiley I'm so damn happy receptionist lady, with full head of hair (Yes, I'm having a great day today) she asks me to take the first door to my left and wait. I will be collected. I feel like an empty milk bottle. I flop (lack of energy you understand, not bad posture) into a chair.

Chatter in the corridor, staff walks towards me. Oh no! I recognize one of the staff, pure pathetic survival techniques kick in (afterwards I can't believe I've done this). I grab a magazine and raise it high, in front of my face. I used to play netball with the staff member coming right past me. Eventually, hearing click clack heels quieten, I get the courage to lower my magazine, there stands my Female Counsellor. Luckily not the Wing Attack player for a team I can't remember the name of just at that moment.

Bald Bird

"Kaye?" ...Counsellor Lady queries. "Yes!" I reply and follow her pink cardiganed back down a maze of corridors to her room.

Well the session goes ok; I find it difficult to let go of my personnel barrier. Well, after all, it has been my inner defence for years, but slowly I start to put out information.

Slowly I give my true feelings of how my life is right now, you know already, so just to say it comes out in blips and blobs. My palms are sweaty by the end of the session.

My Counsellor suggests I look into getting a light hobby or an interest to take my mind off things, meanwhile suggests I book another session for three weeks' time. This will be after my last Chemo, as I'm really nervous about coming off of Chemo. Being left without protection against my own cells that want to attack me.

I leave the building and sit motionless in my car feeling rather stunned with it all. I really need to do something to take my mind off things. We've always wanted a dog.

Bald Bird

Aunty Steff holds the key

My Aunty Steff phones, we chat that evening, she is thinking of getting a Terrier Puppy. Oh, I laugh I would love a Basset Hound. I can remember Nana's Bassett Hound low slung like a lion. Steff laughs, and jokingly offers to buy me one, that's if Mick would be okay with it, we muse. How about a Rescue dog, Steff suggests. This of course is the answer. Steff and I finish our phone call.

"Mick?" Mick agrees to my idea, as do the children, as long as the dog isn't allowed in the front room Mick says. We agree. Anyway, phone Steff the next night, who is ecstatic that Basset Hound a possibility. I receive in the post a few days later a card with a Bassett on and some money to purchase a collar and lead.

Emily and I go to a local dog Sanctuary in Poole. Sadly, no Bassets await us, though plenty of Hienz57, also Greyhounds of all colours. Sadly, we are after the more sluggish side of the market. We are advised to go through a specialist dog rescue and am put in touch with one such lady.

Wendy is in charge of Basset Rescue. she phones me that evening, talking about firstly my illness and if this is a wise decision. she says these dogs are very therapeutic, they make you smile. Also went through how hard work they are, and stubborn. Once the vetting process was discussed, she confirmed that a Home visit would be arranged for Anne to do a Home Check. Anne by the way also bred Bassets.

It was the following evening Anne rang us, asking if it was possible for her to pop round and do the home check, I agreed.

Bald Bird

Long Story short we were approved, much to Emily and George's excitement. Anne leaves us with some Basset books to look at.

A few days later Wendy phones us, saying there is a possibility of a male Bassett coming up for re-homing would we be interested. I'm a bit knocked back as didn't expect such a quick result, and was planning to finish Chemo first, however having spoken with mum, Mick, and children, decide we would like to see him.

Emily and George stay with mum, the thought process being that if the dog wasn't a good fit, they would find it hard to leave him behind. Mick finds Wendy's house, and outside are a pack of Bassets varying in size and colour. I spot a beauty, he's massive but his tail doesn't stop wagging. Actually, that was the dog for re-homing!

Barney was soon ours having signed, micro chipped, gone through Eukenuba feed, and Ear Drops. With a bit of help lifting his rear into the car Barney was ours. Looking at him in the mirror with his ears blowing back looked like he was smiling, all that was needed to complete the look was goggles.

Home. Mum opens the door, and gasps at Barney's length. She thinks he's more like a crocodile, Barney doesn't wait to be invited in, he hurtles past into the waiting arms - squeals of delight - of Ems and George. They think he's great. As do we all. Apart from the cat.

Bald Bird

4th Chemo, 05.04.00

Following 4th Chemo, Mick takes me home after asking if vitamin supplements are a good idea, the doctor is positive about this but says be careful and not to overdo things, this had been a gruelling session. Each session makes me feel weaker.

Mum sits for us in the evening so we can go out for a few hours. Luckily, the weather is still cold, and I can justify wearing a woolly hat. We have a lovely evening. Mick knocks back a few pints; I drink Orange juice and am designated driver.

Bald Bird

5th Chemo, 03.05.00

I'm really pleased with my progress and am beginning to start planning things following Chemo. I wait for Dr Dean to give the all clear for my regime to begin. But unfortunately, that doesn't happen. My blood count is to bloody low. I remember that woman on my first appointment and I feel all her frustration. But hell, what can you do but just accept. It means I wouldn't finish treatment till end of May; my hair wouldn't start growing till middle of June...hey hang on here, I'm being optimistic!

I amaze myself. And with this make my appointment and leave with Mick.

Mick suggests booking us a holiday. We walk slowly round the shops in Weymouth, I feel like an old lady in a young person's body. Thinking of laying on a warm beach sounds like heaven.

Staring in shop windows we see a few deals and go in and ask for details. We then ask if the package entails health insurance, something we can't travel without I remind Mick. This brings us down to earth with a bang. £500.00 for a week. I say forget it lets just go to Gould's Garden centre for a mooch round, tea, coffee, and some cake.

Sitting in the garden I exhale and just enjoy not feeling sick or dizzy. Mick has gone quiet. He's up to something. I follow his gaze, as he sips his coffee that follows a path to second-hand caravans.

Having finished our drinks, we follow the path to caravan heaven. Some are expensive but tucked up in the far corner is a little gem - just brought in on a Trade Up. A four berth Winetta.

Bald Bird

The Salesman came over for a chat, saying she was just in and needs cleaning, but would we like to take a look? "Yes" says Mick. Key found - we enter caravan. Dusky pink lounge carpet. Four berths in good order. Double bed at backroom. Tidy kitchen and working loo. Mick buys it then and there for £400.00.

Winnie the caravan joins our family. That evening Mick calls round work colleagues, looking for storage for Winnie. A farmer in Chickerell rents a field problem solved. The following weekend we go to Durdle Door with all the kids. The great outdoors. Caravanning is great, we play cricket, tennis, walk the dog, eat lots, and play cards during the evening, before bed.

All too soon the weekend's over, time to pack up and leave the caravan field, that only as us and one other caravan.

Bald Bird

My last Chemo, 24.05.00

I have had my last chemo. I've done it, my families done it yippee! I thank all the nurses for their never-ending support. Jean and I arrange to meet in six months and promise to keep in touch by phone. We hug.

 My last Chemo, I am so anxious not to be having more of these Cancer cell busting- wonder drugs, that cease my cells to develop in mad patterns, build, multiply and multiply.

I phone a Breast Buddy- A breast Buddy is someone post treatment, who voluntarily links up with the NHS to support newly diagnosed patients.

My Buddy is Fran, she is two years post treatment, and lives just down the road on Portland. Fran knows and recognises my fears, concerns and where I'm coming from.

Fran is calming; she tells me we are ultimately in charge of our bodies, that the Chemo stays in our bodies for a long time, continuing its job of killing Cancer cells. I would also be having three monthly check ups for the first year, and mammograms yearly, umm... a little bit calmer now. We Chat about our families, and then about my return to work.

Fran is now back to work full time. I'm planning to go back September. Firstly, though we have the children's six-week summer holiday. I will use this time to re cooperate. Good idea Fran says, don't rush back before you feel really well. We say goodbye and good lucks.

Jean supports me, responding swiftly to my panicky messages, when I find numerous lumps and bumps everywhere which in reality, have always been present but due to my constant checks only now discovered.

I join the local Breast Care Support Group, as advised by Jean that is held in a church hall in Weymouth, there is a lady there that had a Mastectomy 20 years ago, also a lady that has Secondaries.....I also meet another lady called Mary, we become friends and arrange to meet. She had a Mastectomy five years ago. If anyone walked into this room now, they would almost question if they were in a keep fit class the way people are so bubbly.

Bald Bird

Getting back to life

The summer holidays fly by, we enjoy hot sunny days down the beach, picnics.

For me searching out a shady spot, I am sporting a new swimming costume; the top is like a bikini sports top, covers down to my ribs. I am aware of the red scar on my back, my life scar I have called it.

We build sandcastles and enjoy just being. George gets into a very large sand fight, Mick has to intervene, as sun bathers are getting covered, little sods. George comes back looking like a sandman. Ice cream is bought, and everyone settles back down.

All the girls are making sand mermaids, using seaweed for hair. The sky is blue and the sea gently laps, life is good, no life is brilliant. I look at my family and sigh content just in that moment.

The holidays are coming to a close; my children have had a great time being generally

spoiled, by family and friends. They seem very strong little people now; they are more independent of me, more self-sufficient. Mick continues going to work, seeing his girls.

My beloved mum has at last had the news her drains are now sorted in her house, and she can shortly return home. That will feel strange I've got used to her being around.

Bald Bird

Back to work

Holidays are over, its September. School gates creak open, and swarms of children sway up the street on the path back to education. They pretend not to be happy about this as they chat excitedly to reunited friends that they have missed over the hols.

Emily and George have gone, the house is empty apart from Barney and me. I can even hear the mantle clock ticking. I sit and have a coffee, having tidied away

Breakfast dishes go upstairs to get my work shoes. I pause and look at my reflection; I wonder how my colleagues will react to my return. I have gained a little weight now, and my hair is now short and wavy, darker than my Strawberry blonde before.

I put Barney out in his kennel, check he has clean water.

"Well Barney, this is it, I'm back to work!" Barney lays down on his blanket looking at me quizzically. Walking back through the kitchen to the hall I pick up the keys from their hook.

Stop, turn round, and take a last look. I thought this day would never come.

Driving to work I feel the rush of exhilaration.

I am away from home. I'm going to work!

Arriving in Dorchester, drive around for five minutes; trying desperately to find a parking spot (Always difficult in a hospital car park). I have to give up and decide to try further afield. Cutting down the back streets, I turn into Dagmar Road. That is where I lived with my first husband, Emily and George's Dad. Gosh, that seems a lifetime ago. I park up, pause, and smile. I slip through the back alley to Williams Avenue and cross the

Bald Bird

main road. Before I go to the main hospital. I pop in and say hello to one of the secretaries in The Children's Centre.

After I walk up the steps towards the Pencils (Large mobile of different coloured pencils-Some Architects dream) turn left and get lift up to Hardy Ward. Pass the large photos of staff. "Hello, it's good to be back." I say this quietly as I pass by.

Balloons are attached to our office door. I enter "Welcome back!" banners go across the room; more balloons are attached to the walls. I see a card for me, signed from Natalie, Karyn, and Claire.

I turn then get into my in tray.

Life slips to normality.

However, I find that after a while working in a hospital environment is challenging. Feeling the need to change direction workwise, I look into doing a Reflexology Course at the Weymouth College: A Holistic Course.

Ringing up, I find the course is 3 weeks in but if I feel ok about it, they have one space. Passing the interview, I grab the course! The course is one day a week (Perfect) and will fit in with my working hours. I'm rather proud of my whites, looking like someone from a Daz Advert. I have also decided that I want to change my job, I have always enjoyed working with the Elderly and would like to go back to working in the community.

After many walks with mum at Abbotsbury along the beach path (This is where we always churned things over) debating should I, shouldn't I give up my hospital job, I decide to do just that. I have learnt such a lot in this job, and the characters I have met I will never forget. Especially my very first patient Jimmy.

Bald Bird

Following his Stroke all he could say was the F word. But every Christmas Jimmy sent me a Christmas card.

Natalie and Karyn were sad I was leaving but understood and wished me well in my new position with Carewey. I had got a job with an elderly lady and her son who lived six doors up from me. Couldn't have worked out better.

Time ticks by, the children relax; mum is well settled back in her house now.

Barney lolls around the house. Rabbits sunbathe in the garden. Pickles, well she's just the same, sneaking in with the Guinea pigs.

We all regain our independence. I catch up with friends that found my illness difficult to cope with. Emily and George have as many friends round as we can pack in. I can recognise who's there by the trainers in the hall.

I relish not having to drive to work and enjoy making new work friends.

Through "Bosom Buddies", a Support group I joined, I meet Monica who lives on Portland just round the corner from me, she also works for "Weymouth and Portland Housing".

Monica asks if I would like to apply for a part time cleaning post at Ladymead Hall.

I go for the interview but am offered not the cleaning job but a Wardens position starting in February, it's all happening!

Emily's loft conversion is now complete- Ems takes up new residency. George switches rooms and paints his room with Mick. Yes, Orange and red again. Complete with new bunk bed and

Bald Bird

desk underneath. Kitty and Sally have their bunk beds in George's old room,

Health check-ups pass well, 1 month, then 3 months.

Then it's Christmas. Mick cooks, and we all celebrate. What a year!

Feb, March slip by, April, May, June and then July & at last I qualify as a Reflexologist!!!! Whoopee doo!

Now I work occasionally (voluntarily having got through the vetting process) as a Reflexologist for Hamwick House, treating Cancer patients. This is, as and when required. It's the least I can do after all. Now I can give something back to the NHS as a thank you for all the care I received.

Not the end!

Bald Bird

2020

2020 - I am completing this journal twenty years after being diagnosed with Grade 3 Breast cancer.

I am 54 years old, happily married, children grown and Grandchildren, mum is well and reliable as ever! Have my own Dog Grooming Salon - Hair Off The Dawg - working from home. Alive and well with no reoccurrence 20 years on from first being diagnosed with Grade 3 Breast cancer. I'm alive!

I never thought I would say this, but I have been so very lucky. I have a loving family, Mum -Old Reliable, Andy and children and now Grandchildren .

Never ever be frightened to get help and support for this - I requested yearly Mammograms rather than every three years - which the NHS supported me with. I truly struggled with the fear of the disease returning.

Mental Health – Important - I have continued to use and will always use/have the support of Counselling Via my GP, Anti-Depressants/medication if and when needed. And, of course, if I'm worried about any lump or bump, I scuttle off swiftly and get it checked out by my GP! Who are eternally patient with me, and will be with you.

My life has gone through massive lows, and highs. A rollercoaster ride of emotions.

I met and Married Andy who is my soul mate, bringing to the fold his two sons - we have been married ten years this year, thank you so much for your never ending patience and support of me and our expanding family. Now lovingly known as Grandy to our grandchildren.

Bald Bird

Emily my beautiful daughter married Darren, they have two beautiful, healthy, happy children. Thankyou Emily for making my dreams come true, making me a Grandma and Andy a Grandy - we are truly blessed.

George is now grown up, relocated with Andy and Me eventually to Worcester and has recently purchased and lives with his much-wanted German Shepherd Nikolai (21st Birthday present) in his one-bedroom house, wahoo! Working at a local Homeless Hostel as a Support Worker. So proud of you love.

RIP –Barney, Pickles, and the Guinea pigs. (We miss you still) - Rip Charlie my Chocolate Springador dog, 9 years old (Shoe-pincher, and the lazy lump in my bed!).

Hello to Jack the Jack Russell and Pablo, a Chihuahua.

Hello to my new career working from home as a Dog Groomer.

Bald Bird

Thank You

Thankyous, where do I begin?

Emily and George for all you went through, all your support love and cuddles, I love you forever.

Mum - Old Reliable - Wow what a trooper for your never-ending care, love and support. You were there for us as always. We love you so much.

Gran and Grandad. We lost Grandad a few years ago and we miss you dreadfully.

Aunty Steff, Danny, Davina for all your phone calls and visits. Thank you.

Last, but by no means least, my lovely new husband Andy who I met at Weymouth and Portland Housing Christmas do 2004. Andy, you mean so much to me. You light up my life with love, laughter and kindness. We got married at Gretna Green on 31st July 2010. I love you so much, especially when your eyes twinkle!

I'm Alive!!!!!

Dorchester County Hospital Thank you for the gift of extended life.

Mr Consultant, Jean, all the nurses and all the wonderful women who I met along the way.

Thank you.

To my Bosom Buddy friend Fran who sadly passed away.

To Monica, Bosom Buddy friend were doing well aren't we! xxxx

Printed in Great Britain
by Amazon